"As a Member of Co   s
to the problems our co
health care crisis and de
of their health care deci: ...other example
of the excellent work the   ...gton Policy Center produces."

-Congresswoman Cathy McMorris Rodgers
(5th District, Washington state)

"Dr. Stark's cogent analysis of America's health care challenges takes the thoughtful, incisive approach of a surgeon and combines it with the well-researched arguments of an experienced public policy analyst. A most worthwhile read for anyone interested in both a diagnosis of and prescription for our Nation's health care ills."

-Washington State Attorney General Rob McKenna

"Roger Stark thoroughly captures the story of health care in America in a studious but highly readable style. His outstanding book will stimulate understanding and concrete solutions to one of the most critical issues of our time. It is essential reading for all who care about sustaining quality health care in the United States."

-Former Congressman George R. Nethercutt, Jr.
(5th District, Washington state)

"Dr. Stark's book is a treasure, explaining accurately, clearly, and concisely how we have reached the current state of 'Health Care in the United States Today' and offering common sense solutions to the problems we face. His years of experience in the health care system as a cardiac surgeon give him a valuable perspective on what works and what doesn't work in our health sector. He offers a concise explanation of the problems we face, the history behind how we got here, what other countries have done to their health systems, and solutions that make ethical and economic sense for America. This second edition also explains the terrible damage that Obamacare will do to what has been the finest health care in the world. No matter how much you know about health care in America, there is much to be learned here. Dr. Stark shines a beacon of light on the right path to replace Obamacare with sensible policies that will work for America."

-Grace-Marie Turner
President, Galen Institute

THE PATIENT-CENTERED SOLUTION

Our Health Care Crisis, How It Happened,
and How We Can Fix It

Second edition of
Health Care In the U.S. Today:
Problems and Solutions (2007)

ROGER A. STARK M.D.

CONTENTS

THE PATIENT-CENTERED SOLUTION:
OUR HEALTH CARE CRISIS, HOW IT HAPPENED, AND HOW WE CAN FIX IT

SECOND EDITION OF
HEALTH CARE IN THE U.S. TODAY:
PROBLEMS AND SOLUTIONS (2007)

By Roger Stark, MD, FACS

PREFACE

I have worked in medicine my entire adult life, first as a busy cardiovascular and thoracic surgeon and, after retirement from active practice, as the executive director of a hospital foundation and a health care policy analyst for a major state-based think tank. During my career, I worked at over twenty hospitals and dealt with insurance companies, health maintenance organizations, Medicare, Medicaid and the uninsured. I have run for both federal and state office and have firsthand knowledge of the political process.

This book started as an op-ed piece on health care reform for a local newspaper. While organizing my thoughts, I quickly realized that defining the problems with our current health care system and explaining the solutions was impossible within the allotted 600 word limit. On the other hand, I think it is accurate to say that few people outside the academic world would read a three to four hundred page policy book on the subject.

Consequently, I wrote this short book. My purpose is to provide a concise explanation of our health care crisis, the history behind it, our treatment alternatives and the solutions that make the most ethical and economic sense for the United States.

Health care has changed dramatically over the past one hundred years. Most U.S. citizens have a general idea of what is right and what is wrong with our current medical care delivery system, but most people lack a clear understanding of the various factors that add to our health care crisis and the history that got us to this crisis point.

Many people believe the government can solve all the problems by instituting a single-payer, socialized system. Unfortunately, the single-payer system has not made economical sense in other countries and is the exact opposite of virtually all other economic interactions in the United States. Only when patients can act as true consumers and can control their own health care will we be able to solve our current crisis in medical care delivery.

I hope you, the reader, reach the final chapter with a clear grasp of our health care system's history and problems, and understand why I believe the solutions I propose make sense for our country. Though much longer than that op-ed piece I started out to write, I included only those facts and developments crucial to understanding our current situation.

Roger Stark, MD, FACS
2007

PREFACE TO THE SECOND EDITION

A tremendous amount has happened in health care since the First Edition was published in 2007. The passage of the Patient Protection and Affordable Care Act (PPACA) in March, 2010, was a real game-changer for health care in the United States. If fully implemented, the new law will be as significant as the passage of Medicare and Medicaid in 1965. The PPACA was passed by a strict partisan vote. Never before in the history of the U.S. has such a major piece of social legislation become law without the support of both political parties.

Although the vast majority of Americans believe health care reform is necessary, over 50 percent of people continue to want the PPACA repealed and replaced. I have devoted an entire chapter to the new legislation. Unless repealed, the law will push this country much further toward centrally-planned, government-controlled health care. The decisions and wishes of patients and providers will have much less importance than the plans of the government.

The passage of PPACA makes this book all the more relevant in the ongoing health care debate in the U.S.

I would like to thank Paul Guppy, Vice President for Research, and John Barnes, Communications Director, at the Washington Policy Center for their input and assistance with this Second Edition.

Roger Stark, MD, FACS

2012

1.
INTRODUCTION

Let's talk about food. I know this is a book about health care, but let's begin by looking at some of the aspects of, for lack of a better term, "food care".

I think we can all agree that food is a necessary requirement for a long, productive, happy life. People eat varying amounts of food and some individuals have specific nutritional requirements. In general, nearly everyone in this country has enough to eat. Not everyone can afford caviar or steak every day and, fortunately, government welfare and charities are there to help those who can't afford the basics. Eating permeates our society and, including restaurants, food is a multi-billion dollar industry. There are essentially no food shortages in the United States. Although we have an entire government department for agriculture, complete with some crop subsidies and other various programs, the free market works pretty well in providing food for everyone.

So what is different about health care compared to food care? For starters, everyone knows we must eat every day, but no one knows for sure when each of us will need health care.

Fair enough, but unless we are in complete denial, we all realize that at some point we will probably need some type of medical intervention. I mean, everybody has taken an aspirin, sprained some body part, or knows someone who needed to see a doctor or go to a hospital.

Okay, you say, but food care is a pay-as-you-go system where groceries are expensed out every week or month, and eating at that local restaurant (fancy or not) is included in the family budget somewhere. If you don't have a lot of money this week, you don't buy the steak. One grocery store has a better deal on green beans, so you shop there. If you can't afford the best restaurant, take the family out for fast food. Whatever is required for your food care needs – be it more food or more specialized food - you have choices that allow you to buy the foods you need.

So what about health care? Can't budget for it now? Don't want to budget for it now? Don't know how to budget for it? Sadly to say, you probably can't. Not that you are not smart enough or concerned enough. It is simply that our current health care system is broken and will not allow you to purchase medical care as you can food care.

But, health care is much more expensive than food care, you claim. Plus, you never exactly know when you might need it. It is sort of like paying for car or home repair after a crash or after some catastrophe, isn't it? Of course, what allows us to deal with this expensive, unpredictable auto or home event is a viable, competitive and relatively free market system of auto and home insurance. For routine vehicle and home maintenance, we pay as we go. Yet for those expensive and infrequent events, we rely on our various insurance policies to cover costs after the deductible.

Let's get back to food. Although the U.S. constitution does not say so, I think we would all agree that everyone in this country has a "right" to food care. Of course, that does not mean that you can walk into your local grocery store and steal food off of the shelves. It does mean government exists to provide citizens an open market for the delivery and purchase of food. It also means that if you cannot afford food, you can still have access to it by applying for government food stamps or by taking advantage of the various charity programs in your community.

Unfortunately, my analogy of food versus health care breaks down at this point, because the people of this country cannot access medical care in a free and open market as they can food. This lack of access to health care is a direct result of the way our health care system has developed since the turn of the twentieth century.

We are faced with a health care system that is doomed to fail. Although we now enjoy the most sophisticated medical care ever known, we absolutely cannot sustain the massive costs of the system we have built to provide this medical care. Health care expenses continue to rise each year at a rate nearly double our gross domestic product (GDP). If our health care system continues to run as it currently does, by the year 2030 we will spend 11 percent of our GDP on Medicare and Medicaid alone (Ezrati 2004), and mathematics suggest that at the same rate by 2050 we will spend fully one third of our GDP on medical care. From a basic economic standpoint, this scenario is not sustainable.

Figure 1
National Health Expenditures as a Percentage of
Gross National Product (GNP) and
Gross Domestic Product (GDP)
1929-2010

Virtually no one in this country is happy with our current system. Employers are paying more each year for employee health benefits; employees are paying a higher deductible in most cases; the poor are finding it more difficult to access health care; the elderly are paying more and finding their choices of physicians and hospitals more limited; hospitals are dealing with declining reimbursement; health care workers are grappling with job dissatisfaction and decreasing compensation; and certain specialty care is limited in many communities. Many physicians are looking for a career change or are taking early retirement. Interestingly, their decreasing satisfaction has nothing to do with diminishing income, but it does have to do with decreasing autonomy and less ability to provide high-quality care, and a loss of their ability to manage their time with patients.

What I intend to show in this book is how we have gradually arrived at this disastrous point, what the future alternatives are, and what makes the most medical, ethical, and economic sense to correct our current health care crisis. A massive overhaul of virtually all aspects of the health care system will be required – but bear with me, and remember that health care is no more necessary than food care.

At the end of the day, health care is really about the relationship between patients and their medical care providers and in no way needs to be as complex as it has become. Just as virtually everyone understands how to provide food and shelter for themselves and their families, so too can everyone understand how to obtain and evaluate their health care.

Unlike most books on health care policy, this one is designed to provide a broad overview in a brief, easily readable and reasonably short form. I intend to show that patients have the most interest in their own medical care and that consumer-driven medicine is the only reasonable answer to our current health care dilemma.

2.
HISTORY

So how did we get into this health care crisis? What historically set us up for the problems we now face? Like so many things, we can get a better understanding of our current problems by knowing the crucial steps, and missteps, that the country took along the way. In general, each new law or regulation or program made sense at the time it was enacted, but it was not necessarily made in the context of our overall health care system. There was no master plan or overall design as health care developed in the United States. Multiple political agendas, pressures from the choices other countries were making, and an accepted philosophy that health care is a right to which we are all entitled led to our medical system developing much differently than that of any other service or commodity in the United States.

The history of health care can be divided chronologically in any number of ways. To simplify things and to use several logical milestones, let's look at three periods; pre-Depression, 1930-1965, and the 1960s up to passage of the Patient Protection and Affordable Care Act in March 2010.

THE PERIOD BEFORE THE GREAT DEPRESSION

There were a number of colonial and then state-sponsored programs that provided care for specific groups and communities in the 1600 and 1700s. The first significant federal program was the 1799 passage of the Act for Relief of Sick and Disabled Seamen. This program became the U.S. Marine Service and, ultimately, at the turn of the twentieth century, became what we now know as the U.S. Public Health Services (USPHS).

Originally, the USPHS managed quarantine issues and the funding of medical research. In the early 1900s, the agency grew to include school health and vaccinations, and received federal funding to operate multiple health clinics throughout the United States. The next one hundred years saw this organization expand tremendously, with an annual budget approaching $100 billion by the end of the twentieth century. Today, the USPHS is involved in several social issues such as cigarette smoking, alcohol abuse, family planning, as well as management of the Indian Health Service.

Congress established the National Academy of Sciences in 1863 to study health care issues nationwide. In 1879, the National Board of Health was created specifically to control epidemics. On the local front, aseptic and antiseptic practices were not only becoming common, but were reassuring people that hospitals were safe and really could heal the sick. From 1873 to 1923, the number of hospitals in the U.S. grew from

178 to 6,830, most of which were built by charities and religious organizations.

The American Medical Association (AMA) was formed in the mid-nineteenth century to promote safe medicine and to protect the interests of patients and doctors. From the beginning, however, the AMA was heavily politicized and its leaders had very definite ideas concerning appropriate medical practice. It opposed physicians contracting with fraternal lodges because of "ruinous competition" (Contract Practice 1907) and refused membership into county medical societies to those doctors that did contract their services. Likewise, the AMA opposed and fought physicians' participation in pre-paid health care, which had become common with large companies in dangerous industries such as mining and logging.

By the end of the nineteenth century, health care was already divided along national lines and private or charity offerings. Most citizens at that time believed the federal government should participate in major health issues such as epidemiology, the study of the spread of disease. For local, routine care - seeing the doctor or going to a hospital - most people believed in using the private system.

Internationally, however, the socialist and labor movements lobbied heavily for nationalized health care during the late nineteenth and early twentieth centuries. Germany, in 1883, became the first country to formally provide comprehensive state-run medicine. In the U.S., the Socialist Party pushed for socialized medicine in the 1904 presidential election, and the Progressive Party of Theodore Roosevelt made socialized medicine a campaign issue in 1912.

At that same time, twelve state legislatures considered bills for compulsory health care and more than one governor expressed support for the concept.

By World War I, more than ten European countries had socialized their medical care systems. Enthusiasm for socialized health care in the U.S., however, waned tremendously after the war because of its negative association with Germany and Russia. Voters were also smart enough to realize there was no real need to socialize their medical care. No state passed any form of government-run health care, and only sporadic interest existed on a national level. While charities and religious groups built the hospitals, fraternal orders and lodges offered their members a form of health and life insurance. Probably less than 10 percent of the country had any type of personal health insurance during the early twentieth century.

As lines were being drawn over who was providing what type of care, physician training was also coming under considerable scrutiny at the beginning of the twentieth century. In 1910, the Carnegie Foundation commissioned a study to examine physician education in the U.S. The result of this study, the Flexner Report, recommended state licensing of graduates from qualified medical schools only. Prior to this report, medical training was offered at various types of schools, with no standardized graduation requirements and no assurance of quality. The number of medical schools in this country subsequently dropped from 131 to 69 in the next 34 years, care became more standardized and quality of care improved.

The 1920s saw an extension of veterans' benefits after World War I. Congress established the Veterans Bureau in 1921, and by 1929 several of these programs were consolidated into the Department of Veterans Affairs.

On an international scope, Europe was rebuilding after World War I, and the nationalization of health care became commonplace.

Basically, life was good in the U.S. during the 1920s - we had won the Great War, the economy was booming, unemployment was low and health care was not an issue for most people. Interestingly enough, however, the first comprehensive study of the U.S. health care system was undertaken in 1927. A small group of national leaders, including many physicians, formed the Committee on the Costs of Medical Care (CCMC), which was funded by eight philanthropic foundations. In spite of widespread opposition to socialized medicine in the U.S., the CCMC recommended a long-range plan for instituting national health care. Unfortunately the committee did not even determine, or attempt to estimate, how many people actually lacked access to health care in this country, nor did it estimate a cost for socializing medicine in the U.S.

Although the CCMC cannot be faulted for failing to predict the technological explosion in health care in the twentieth century, it was totally irresponsible of the committee not to put some type of price tag on socializing medicine in the U.S. Unfortunately, this became a recurring theme as the twentieth century unfolded, where need, predicted benefit and ultimate cost were, if not totally ignored, at least not emphasized in government intervention in health care in this country.

THE GREAT DEPRESSION TO 1960

When the economy went into a tailspin in 1929, the medical sector was not immune to the crash. The average hospital reimbursement dropped from $200 per patient in 1929 to $60 per patient in 1930 (Califano, 1986, p. 41).

Patients, providers and hospitals were caught up in the financial uncertainties of the 1930s. The U.S. saw the institution of prepaid health care as a partial answer to the financial insecurity. In 1929, 1,500 school teachers at Baylor University Hospital in Dallas, Texas, started the first group insurance plan. In 1932,

Blue Cross as we know it today was started by multiple hospitals in the Sacramento, California area. These programs provided prepaid health care on a group basis and were called medical, or health care, insurance. From the onset, these plans were not truly "insurance" in the classic sense, but rather prepaid health "maintenance" programs in that they covered everything from routine care, such as annual exams, or "maintenance," to emergency care and other unplanned and unexpected needs for health care – those health events comparable to car insurance covering accidents and homeowners insurance covering fires. This concept of maintenance rather than insurance has survived and has become the accepted definition of health "insurance." It is a colossal misnomer in health care discussions. By 1940, there were multiple prepaid health plans throughout the country, as well as two large health maintenance organizations, the Kaiser Industry Program and the Group Health Association. All were providing coverage for health maintenance care.

As the 1930s progressed, Blue Cross enlarged as it covered hospital expenses, and Blue Shield emerged and expanded to cover physician reimbursement. From a political standpoint, the AMA strongly opposed health maintenance organizations and prepaid plans other than Blue Cross and Blue Shield. The "Blues" were heavily supported by organized medicine and retained that support throughout the twentieth century.

The 1930s saw a huge expansion of both state and federal intervention into many aspects of the U.S. economy, including the health care delivery system. The Ransdell Act of 1930, for example, greatly enlarged the National Institute of Health. Although President Roosevelt was extremely interested in nationalizing health care as part of his New Deal, he never lobbied strongly for it, using the excuse that it was impossible to go up against the medical societies. In reality, however, a massive voter revolt forced Congress to remove the national health care provision from the Social Security legislation of 1935 (Feingold 1966, pp.91-92). The majority of people believed they had satisfactory access to health care and did not want the federal government to control their relationships with doctors and hospitals. On the state level, all but four states had compulsory workers' compensation programs in place. Interestingly, in addition to most Americans being satisfied with their health care in the early 1930s, health care at this time accounted for approximately four percent of the GDP, a reasonable and acceptable sum (Harris 1966, p.9).

The controversy over national social insurance specifically for retirement, in other words Social Security, was taken as high as the Supreme Court. The Court ruled in 1937, in Hekvering v. Davis, that the concept of a mandatory socialized insurance program was constitutional. That decision laid legal groundwork, but again, there was no widespread enthusiasm for the institution of socialized medical insurance in the U.S. at that time.

By 1940, as the debate over nationalizing health insurance continued, Blue Cross had grown to six million members and commercial insurance had approximately 3.7 million subscribers. Although Blue Cross and commercial insurance carriers were direct competitors, they had several distinct differences. Blue Cross, by law, did not have to hold reserves, had very significant tax advantages, and had no minimum benefit or premium rates. These are advantages that Blue Cross has maintained in various forms down through the years.

As the 1940s unfolded, the health care insurance industry had become fairly mature. Again, it cannot be stressed enough that health "insurance" is clearly different than other forms of true indemnity insurance. Unlike car and home policies that do not cover routine maintenance, health policies are designed to cover routine medical care as well as unplanned occurrences.

Also of significance is the fact that doctors were paid through a usual and customary fee arrangement, whereas hospitals were paid on a "cost plus" basis. This was a very convoluted plan which reimbursed hospitals not for a specific service, but on a percentage of their total costs as well as on a percentage of the number of policyholders of any one company using that hospital. Larger hospitals were reimbursed at a higher percentage rate than smaller hospitals. This led to a disincentive for hospitals to control costs, since higher reimbursements followed higher expenditures. This bizarre arrangement continues to a minor degree today and is simply one more piece of the health care crisis puzzle.

World War II brought about many changes in this country, not the least of which was how the federal government impacts people's lives. The U.S. income tax rate increased from four percent in 1939 to 23 percent in 1944. In 1940, 14.6 million people filed income tax returns and by 1945, 49.8 million people filed returns, although the population had only increased by six percent (Carson 1977, pp. 124-129). Understandably, there was a war to support, yet, unfortunately, the door had clearly been opened to impose an ever-increasing tax-and-spend mentality in Washington, D.C.

The other massively significant legislation during World War II was the institution of wage and price controls. The government limited how much employers could pay workers. The War Labor Board, however, established a policy where fringe benefits of five percent of wages could be offered to employees. About the same time, the IRS ruled that health insurance purchases for employees could be deducted for tax purposes by the employer as a legitimate cost of doing business.

Obviously, health insurance then became a prime fringe benefit to offer workers. This concept of tax-free employer-provided health care is now firmly entrenched in this country.

Unfortunately, the tax laws have been slanted to allow businesses to deduct health insurance from pre-tax dollars, but until recently, individual purchasers and users of the insurance could not do so. Of course, workers are not required to declare the fringe benefit of health care as income. The statistics for employer-paid health care are very revealing. In 1945, employers paid approximately 10 percent of employee health care. By 1950 that number had jumped to 37 percent, and by 1960, larger companies were paying 100 percent of health benefits for their employees (Wesley 1992).

Enrollment in the hospital-only insurance plans skyrocketed in the last few years of the war from seven million subscribers in 1942 to 26 million subscribers in 1945 (Starr 1982, p. 311). Again, the majority of these people had employer-paid health benefits.

The federal government further entrenched itself in health care when it expanded its veterans' care and established the Veterans Hospital Administration system. By 1945, with 91 hospitals, the Veterans Administration system was the largest single health care delivery system in the U.S.

Americans continued to reject nationalizing health care - a poll in 1946 revealed that only 1 percent of U.S. citizens favored it (Cantril 1951, pp. 442-443) – even as the government proposed incremental plans to adopt it, with senior citizens as the first target group. The federal government failed in its efforts from the 1930s until 1950 to establish a plan that would completely nationalize medical care delivery, but Franklin D. Roosevelt, President from 1932 until his death in 1945, favored such a plan, as did President Truman, who followed him.

In 1946, Congress passed the Hill-Burton Act, requiring hospitals to provide free care for twenty years to people who were unable to pay. The bill provided funding for 500,000 additional hospital beds. Federal money of $4.4 billion was added to the $9.1 billion from state and local taxing agencies to fund the program. The Hill-Burton Act expired in 1978, but clearly set a precedent for substantial government funding of health care.

It can't be emphasized enough that the poor in this country, both seniors and those under sixty five, had access to paid health care through the Hill-Burton Act. Of course, this was a disincentive for many people to buy health insurance, because they knew they would be covered by the government-mandated program. And remember, this was prior to Medicare and Medicaid legislation in 1965.

Another event that caused health care coverage to increase dramatically was the 1948 Labor Relations Board decision that said unions could negotiate for health care benefits for their members. Down through the years, this has become a huge negotiating point for the unions. In 1949, 2.7 million union workers were covered by health care benefits, exploding to 12 million workers by 1955.

Also during the post-World War II years, the National Institute of Health expanded from a budget of $180,000 in 1945, to a budget of $400 million in 1960. The National Science Foundation was also started in 1950 and the Department of Health, Education and Welfare was established in 1953. Again, during the 1950s, the voters understood government funding for broad-based scientific and research organizations, but still opposed any form of socialized medicine.

Although many government interventions into health care took place during the mid twentieth century, four significant landmark acts contributed heavily to our current health care crisis.

First, there is the prepaid insurance model set up during the 1930s. It was very clear from the outset that this was not insurance in the traditional sense, but was in fact a maintenance health care program. This seemed advantageous to patients as well as to hospitals and providers at that time, but it set a lasting precedent for what we expect health insurance to be.

Second, the cost-plus concept of hospital reimbursement basically rewarded expanded care, expensive services and greater utilization, all of which created disincentives to control costs.

Third, the fact that employers could take a business income tax deduction for the cost of employee health benefits definitely entrenched the concept of third-party payers in the latter half of the twentieth century. This originally seemed like a win-win proposition until costs exploded for employers, and employees faced limited access options and higher co-pays. The entire concept of someone else paying for health care was a recipe for over-utilization and, consequently, exploding costs.

Lastly, the Hill-Burton Act firmly entwined federal government funding with state government funding to subsidize the construction of both public and private hospitals. As part of the deal, the nation's poor were provided government-sponsored health care in a regulated, organized fashion. Although you might think this solved the problem of providing health care for the uninsured poor, in reality, it was one of the first steps down the road to socialized medicine.

1960 TO 2010

Although the vast majority of people in the U.S. remained opposed to socialized medicine in the 1950s, President Truman, in office from 1945 until 1953, made several attempts at socializing health care. However, President Eisenhower, who followed him and remained in office until 1961, opposed the idea, and Congress did not seriously consider any health delivery legislation through the mid-to-late 1950s.

The idea of socialized medicine resurfaced when it became a campaign issue in 1960, with President Kennedy favoring a broad-based hospital insurance program through Social Security and President Nixon favoring an expansion of what was later to become the Kerr-Mills law.

By 1960, the majority of employees had health insurance through their employers, and this insurance also covered their families. In addition, veterans were covered for both outpatient medical and hospital care through the VA System, and the Indian Health Services covered the Native American population. It was essentially the poor, the elderly, and the unemployed who were not provided specific health care by a third party. It should be noted, however, that they did have hospital coverage through the Hill-Burton Act, and they had access to health insurance through commercial carriers if they chose to buy it.

From 1952 to 1962, the number of seniors with health insurance actually doubled from 30 percent to 60 percent. Washington, D.C., was still concerned, however, about the low-income senior group. To assist these poorer seniors, the Kerr-Mills law was added to the Social Security Amendments of 1960. This was a landmark bill in the sense that it was a precursor to the 1965 Medicare Act.

The Kerr-Mills law was fairly ingenious in that it was a "means-tested" program. In other words, it provided health care for financially qualified poor seniors based on income. Also, it was a voluntary program, run by the states (although funded by the federal government), and it was actually more generous than Medicare in that it included such things as eyeglasses, prescription drugs and dental care.

So by 1962, at least 60 percent of seniors had individual health care insurance and low-income seniors were taken care of by the Kerr-Mills law. Employees were covered by their employers. There was also a thriving private health insurance market and virtually everyone in the U.S. had access to this market. Charities and county hospital facilities provided care for the poor and indigent through the Hill-Burton Act.

Whether it was simply government bureaucracy or an organized effort to sabotage the Kerr-Mills law, the Health, Education and Welfare Department (HEW) continually stalled reimbursing states for health care utilization through the program. The suspicion at the time was that HEW opposed both the voluntary nature of the program and its means-testing requirement, two features that ran counter to the universal coverage, socialized medicine philosophy.

With President Kennedy's death in 1963, several important things changed in Washington, D.C. First, obviously, Lyndon Johnson, already one of the most powerful political leaders of the time, became President. Second, the Democrats enjoyed a landslide victory in 1964. Third, Johnson's first one hundred days in office were more than a honeymoon period with Congress. There was a considerable amount of guilt over President Kennedy's death and consequently, it seemed that President Johnson and the Democratic Congress were able to pass legislation that Kennedy had supported.

Health care for seniors was one of Kennedy's main interests, and in 1965 Johnson pushed the Medicare Bill through Congress. Interestingly enough, the Medicare Bill was tied to a seven percent increase in Social Security benefits for seniors, the first increase since 1959. Obviously, seniors would be much more likely to support any health care legislation that was combined with an increase in their Social Security reimbursement.

The Republicans at the time favored a program called Better Care, which was essentially a voluntary insurance program funded by deducting $3 a month from Social Security and matched by federal funds. Better Care ultimately became Medicare Part B, covering physician reimbursement.

The AMA favored a program called Elder Care, which was essentially an expanded Kerr-Mills program. Elder Care subsequently became Medicaid, providing federal and state funding for the poor and the disabled.

The driving force behind the inclusion of all three programs was Representative Wilbur Mills (D-Ark.), who was Chairman of the House Ways and Means Committee and somewhat of a political genius. At the end of the day, he appeared to give everyone involved what they wanted, and, hence, we wound up with Medicare Parts A and B, and Medicaid. The passage of Medicare and Medicaid created the largest socialized health care program in the world.

Early Medicare looked great. Seniors were provided with essentially free care, hospitals and doctors were given financial support, and the insurance companies were given the financial benefit of administering the whole program. Not surprisingly, the insurance companies discontinued private individual policies for seniors, and, consequently the free market for senior health insurance collapsed.

When comparing Medicare with the Kerr-Mills law, several glaring differences stand out. First of all, the Kerr-Mills program was voluntary, whereas Medicare was tied with Social Security benefits. If seniors opted out of Medicare, they would then lose their Social Security benefits; this was not true of Kerr-Mills coverage. Second, there was no means testing for Medicare - it included every senior regardless of their financial status. And finally, Medicare was less comprehensive than the Kerr-Mills law. Originally drug benefits, eyeglasses and dental care were not provided with Medicare, though Kerr-Mills included these things. For an in depth discussion of Medicare, see Chapter 7.

At the time Medicare was instituted in 1965, health care made up 5.9 percent of our gross domestic product. Compare this with health care's 17.5 percent share in 2010.

Although the majority of people in the United States favored some type of assistance for seniors, especially low-income elderly, the specifics of the Medicare Bill were a mystery to 75 percent of Americans in 1965 (U.S. Committee on Finance hearings, 1965).

No surprise was the fact that health care demand exploded after passage of the Medicare bill. Basically, free and unlimited health care was the driver behind the massive expansion in utilization. Within several years of passage, the federal government realized they had an out-of-control program on their hands. The wisdom of the day suggested that if this country could only train more doctors and build more hospitals, competition would increase and costs would decrease. Obviously, this was faulty economic thinking and instead, costs skyrocketed.

The last few decades of the twentieth century brought about many new regulatory programs to rein in the costs of health care. But in spite of such tactics as managed care, health maintenance organizations (HMOs), and the scheme of reimbursement by diagnosis (diagnostic related group, or DRG, rather than specific treatments), health care costs continued to spiral out of sight in the latter part of the twentieth and first part of the twenty-first centuries.

3.
THE PATIENT PROTECTION AND AFFORDABLE CARE ACT (PPACA)

THE PASSAGE

The most recent debate on health care reform began shortly after the 2008 National Election. Democrats controlled both houses of Congress with wide majorities, as well as the White House.

Although 85 percent of the American public believed the economy and jobs were the most important problems facing the country during the recession of 2009, Congress elected to make health care the major debate of the session. The House of Representatives passed a sweeping health care reform bill in the summer of 2009, and the Senate eventually passed its bill on Christmas Eve. Both bills essentially passed along strict party lines with a significant number of House Democrats in opposition. Likewise, both bills passed by the absolutely slimmest majorities – 218 votes in the House and 60 votes in the Senate to end debate, the bare minimum needed for passage.

Under the normal process for major social legislation, both bills would have gone to a House/Senate conference committee to work out differences and formalize the language. Then the conference committee bill would go back to each house for approval. After passage by both houses, the conference committee bill would go to the President to be signed into law.

However, between the Christmas Eve passage and the first conference committee meeting, Massachusetts held a special election to fill Senator Ted Kennedy's seat. Scott Brown, a Republican who ran against the proposed health care reform bills, was elected. This election reduced the number of Democrats in the Senate from 60 to 59. The Democrats at that point did not have enough votes to pass a conference committee bill and consequently the House simply passed the unamended Senate bill. This was an example of politics at its worst. Up to that point it had been unthinkable that Congress would pass major social legislation affecting one sixth of the U.S. economy on the narrowest of party-line votes.

OVERVIEW OF THE LAW

The final bill as signed by the President was called the Patient Protection and Affordable Care Act (PPACA) and contains over 2800 pages and creates over 160 new government agencies and organizations. By contrast, the Medicare and Medicaid legislation contained less than 200 pages and passed with broad bipartisan majority support.

For the first ten years, PPACA forces ten years of new taxes starting in 2010, but allows for only six years of payout in major benefits starting in 2014. The budget for the first ten years is estimated by the Congressional Budget Office (CBO) to be around $1 trillion. There are no CBO estimates for the second ten years, but independent analyses reveal a potential cost of over $2 trillion, with a substantial burden on the U.S. deficit and ongoing debt.

The funding for the PPACA comes from two main sources. Almost one half of the $1 trillion will come from the largest tax increase the U.S. has ever experienced outside of war years. Taxes will be levied on individuals, employers, drug and medical device manufacturers and insurance companies. The other one half of the $1 trillion will come from massive cuts in Medicare. These cuts are essentially an accounting trick and will simply transfer funding from an existing government health care program to the new health care programs in the PPACA law.

After removing $40-50 billion for administrative costs, the balance of the $1 trillion will essentially fund two programs – a huge expansion of Medicaid ($450 billion) and taxpayer subsidies for people to purchase health insurance in the newly-created state health insurance exchanges ($450-500 billion). These numbers are simply guesses, because no one knows how many people will be eligible for, and claim, the new entitlements.

The reality is that government estimates for costs of entitlements have been universally incorrect and much too low.

SPECIFICS OF PPACA
THE INDIVIDUAL MANDATE

The law is based on an individual mandate that requires every adult in the U.S. to have government-approved health insurance or pay a fine. Individuals who do not have employer-provided or government-provided health insurance will be forced to purchase their own individual policy. The federal government has never required a citizen to purchase a private product or service as a condition of living in this country. Although probably unconstitutional, the proponents of PPACA have invoked the Commerce Clause in the Constitution as support for the legality of the individual mandate.

THE EMPLOYER MANDATE

PPACA forces employers to provide employees with government approved health insurance or pay a fine. There are complex formulas for determining the size of the company and of the fines to be levied. Ultimately, however, employers will have to decide whether it is financially better to purchase employee health insurance or simply pay the fine.

NEW INSURANCE REGULATIONS

Health insurance companies will face two new regulations. The first requires a company to sell insurance to any person regardless of pre-existing conditions. Essentially this means a person can wait until he becomes sick or injured before purchasing insurance. This concept is called guaranteed issue. The second regulation is everyone will be placed into a community-rated risk pool. There will be modifiers for age and smoking, but, ultimately the young and healthy will pay more and older and sicker people will pay less for health insurance.

STATE INSURANCE EXCHANGES

Every state is now required to establish a state or regional health insurance exchange. The exchange will function as an insurance broker where individuals and small groups can buy health insurance. Federal taxpayer subsidies will be provided in the exchange for people earning between 133 percent and 400 percent of the federal poverty level (FPL). Today 400 percent of the FPL is $88,000 for a family of four. This number will rise to $96,000 in 2016. Pricing and benefit packages in the various exchange plans will be set by the federal government. States are allowed some freedom in the design of the exchange, but ultimately the federal government must approve each state's exchange program.

MEDICAID EXPANSION *(See Chapter 8 for Existing Medicaid)*

Medicaid as it now exists is an entitlement for poor families with children, the disabled, and people who need long term care. It is paid for by state and federal tax dollars in a fifty-fifty ratio. PPACA expands Medicaid to any adult who earns less than 133 percent of the FPL. This new entitlement will be paid for by federal taxpayers for the first three years and ultimately (2020) by a combination of federal tax dollars (90 percent) and state tax dollars (10 percent). The existing Medicaid program is rapidly going broke and enrollees are experiencing severe problems receiving quality health care. Even so, it is estimated PPACA will add 16 to 24 million people to the Medicaid program.

MEDICARE CUTS *(See Chapter 7 for Medicare)*

Medicare, which began in 1965, is a government-run health insurance program for people 65 years of age and older. By 1990, Medicare had exceeded its original budget by nine fold and it currently has an unfunded liability of over $100 trillion. Medicare needs reform to remain solvent. PPACA randomly cuts nearly $580 billion from the existing Medicare program. Most of these cuts will be in the form of a decrease in doctor and hospital reimbursements. Because providers are having difficulty covering their overhead with existing Medicare payments, these new cuts will lead more doctors to leave the program and to increased health care access problems for seniors.

AT LEAST 160 NEW AGENCIES

The bureaucratic complexity of the PPACA is breathtaking. The law creates at least 160 new government agencies, committees and panels to oversee and direct our health care. The legislation gives the Secretary of the Health and Human Services Department essentially dictatorial power over our health care system without the checks and balances of our elected officials. Several of these new agencies will determine what treatments are best for which patients. Cost is not supposed to be a factor in the decision-making process. But with costs exploding out of control, these agencies will most certainly use limited public budgets as a reason for denying care.

PPACA essentially allows the government to control our entire health care system, which makes up one sixth of our economy. PPACA expands the Medicaid entitlement and forces taxpayer subsidies in the insurance exchanges for not only the poor but also the upper middle class. It forces individuals to purchase health insurance and lets the government set prices and benefits in our health care system. PPACA is the largest and most invasive piece of social legislation ever passed in the U.S.

WILL PPACA WORK?

In 2005, ten percent of the people in Massachusetts had no health insurance. That year Governor Mitt Romney, a Republican, and the Democratic legislature passed comprehensive health care reform.

The fundamentals of the reform were: an individual mandate requiring everyone not covered by his or her employer to purchase health insurance or pay a fine; an employer mandate to purchase employee health insurance or pay a fine; insurance "reforms" of guaranteed issue and community rating; expansion of Medicaid and finally; a state-based health insurance exchange, or "connector," with extensive state taxpayer subsidies.

The Massachusetts plan, or RomneyCare, was the blueprint for the PPACA legislation. Examining what has happened in Massachusetts will give us a good idea of what we can expect living under PPACA.

The primary goal of RomneyCare was to provide universal health insurance coverage in the state. This has not happened, although the uninsured rate did drop from ten percent to three percent while over 400,000 people in Massachusetts became newly insured. The number of providers did not increase however. Consequently, demand for health care skyrocketed while access plummeted. Rationing of health care by way of waiting lists occurred. The majority of Massachusetts residents say their quality of health care has suffered with RomneyCare.

Taxpayer costs in the state Connector program exploded and insurance premiums in the individual and small group market have risen faster than the national average. Massachusetts is now experiencing a health care budget deficit of over $1 billion.

Solutions proposed and enacted include imposing new taxes on doctors and hospitals, an increase in the state tobacco tax and new taxes on employers and insurers. The current governor has also proposed capping insurance premium increases and asking the federal government for more health care dollars.

The Massachusetts experience with health care reform should serve as a warning of what we can expect from PPACA. (Yelowitz and Cannon, 2010)

4.
REGULATIONS INTENDED TO
CONTROL COSTS PRIOR TO PPACA

In 1970, the Nixon administration felt managed care would provide the solution for increasing costs. The idea behind managed care was to put patients into heavily regulated organizations that would review all expenditures of both hospitals and doctors.

The Health Maintenance Organization (HMO) Act of 1973 was intended to put managed care into practice, but shortly after its passage it became clear that both patients and physicians were not happy with the lack of choice in the program. Patients who had long-standing relationships with their private doctors were often not allowed to continue that relationship if the physician was not part of their HMO panel.

In the first fifteen years of the program, HMOs expanded from 26 plans with 3 million subscribers to 700 plans with 28 million subscribers. By the mid-1990s, however, it had become obvious that HMOs were doing nothing to hold down the costs of health care, and enrollment has subsequently declined.

In 1972, a professional system was established to encourage physicians to practice safely and efficiently. The Professional Standards Review Organization (PSRO), however, had virtually no positive impact on the way physicians practiced or on the cost of health care in the U.S.

The DRG, or prospective payment system, was started in the mid-1980s to reimburse hospitals and doctors based on a Medicare patient's specific diagnosis. With fixed reimbursement for a designated illness or operation, hospitals found themselves at a marked financial disadvantage. Consequently, many hospitals shifted costs to patients with private coverage to make up the difference between what the government would pay and what would cover the hospitals' overhead. This strategy has not been sustainable, as private insurance companies have likewise ratcheted down their hospital reimbursements.

In spite of its reputation as a free market, our health care system is one of the most heavily regulated industries in this country. Reimbursements for hospitals and doctors are fixed by Medicare, Medicaid, and the insurance carriers. How hospitals and doctors are allowed to deliver care is extensively controlled by the government. The types of care insurance companies must offer its clients are regulated by state bureaucracies. Even the number of medical schools and the number of physicians trained are controlled by government oversight. PPACA will only expand these government regulations and controls.

It is estimated that regulations alone account for 10 percent of all health care costs in the U. S. Another alarming statistic is that regulations make health care unavailable to almost 7.5 million people in our country (Conover 2004).

One of the most sweeping efforts at central planning for health delivery was the National Health Planning and Resource Development Act of 1974. This required states to enact a Certificate of Need (CON) system to control expansion of hospitals and medical procedures. Within ten years it was clear the law did indeed regulate health care, but like PSROs implemented in 1972, it did nothing to hold down costs. It was repealed in 1980, although some states continue to have their own CON programs in place.

Other industries also have government guidelines, but in contrast, they extensively use private certification, consumer reports, and other non-government controls. There is no reason the health industry needs more government oversight than other areas of our economy.

5.
MANDATES

INSURANCE POLICY MANDATES

A very specific and colossal impediment to a free market in health care is the state mandate program for insurance carriers. These mandates require insurance companies to offer policies that cover specific types of health care providers regardless of whether the patient wants or needs that care.

In 1970, there were thirty state mandates in the entire country. There are now more than one thousand. It is estimated 25 percent of the uninsured are priced out of the market because of state mandates. The most ludicrous example of an unnecessary mandate is a twenty-five-year-old single male being required to pay for obstetrical coverage.

Over the past thirty years, as the number of mandates in a state has increased, the cost of individual policies has also increased. Likewise, the number of insurance companies in those states has declined, which further decreases competition and consumer choice.

It makes no sense to have government bureaucrats decide what programs should be included in a person's insurance plan. Unfortunately, the trend in the United States is toward more mandates and government regulations.

One excellent and straightforward solution is to allow inter-state commerce in the health insurance industry, so that companies could sell policies across state borders. Logically, the companies based in states with fewer mandates would potentially be in a more competitive position. This would not only increase competition but would also provide greater patient choice. A recent poll shows 72 percent of Americans favor this solution (Cannon and Tanner 2005), and it is discussed further in "Solutions," Chapter 17.

The cost of each mandate varies, but it is estimated that a mandate adds, on average, 0.5 – 2 percent to the cost of an individual health insurance policy. Consequently, consumers in a state such as Washington with over fifty mandates pay at least 25 percent more per policy than consumers in mandate-free states. It is also estimated that mandates account for 15 percent of this country's overall health care costs. (PriceWaterhouseCooper, 2002)

INDIVIDUAL AND EMPLOYER MANDATES

The PPACA mandates that every adult must buy health insurance and that every employer must pay for employee health insurance.

The federal government has never mandated the purchase of any private product or service, although various states have tried mandating health insurance. Hawaii mandated that every state resident buy health insurance in 1974, yet because of non-compliance, the state's uninsured rate remains virtually the same today.

By comparison, there are 47 states that have mandatory auto insurance. Up to 30 percent of drivers in some of those states still have no insurance and nationwide, 20 percent of all fatal crashes are caused by uninsured motorists. It's difficult to see how mandating health insurance will solve our health care problem.

6.
THE FOOD AND DRUG ADMINISTRATION

Patient safety is used as a reason for much of the regulatory burden, and one of the most regulated areas of health care spending in the U.S. is drug development and sales. The Food and Drug Administration (FDA) oversees this process. In 1965, it took approximately two years to develop a new drug and get it through FDA approval at a regulatory cost of $4 million. By 1989, it took three years at a regulatory cost of $231 million. Today, it takes $800 million with an approval time of greater than fifteen years. It is estimated that the process to get a new drug, discovered in 2003, to the patient by 2015 will cost $1.9 billion.

Figure 2
FDA Regulation: Lives Saved vs. Lives Lost

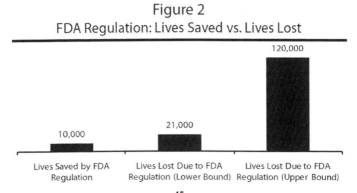

As the FDA ramped up more regulations through the 1970s, with increasing costs to the drug companies and longer processing times, the number of new drugs dropped by almost 60 percent. Obviously this hurt hundreds of thousands of patients who would have been helped by new drug development.

The number of patients experiencing drug side effects can be tracked. The number of patients harmed by not having a drug available is difficult to determine. Consequently, regulators err on the side of drug delay, because drug complications are publishable and reflect on the decision-making process. Although the numbers are difficult to obtain, it is estimated that between 21,000 to 120,000 patients per decade die because of FDA regulations. This is at an estimated cost of $42 billion per year. On the flip side, FDA regulations are estimated to prevent 10,000 deaths per decade at most (Conover 2004).

During the period from 1975-1995, the number of clinical trials mandated for every new drug doubled, and the number of patients required in each trial tripled.

The increasing cost and time of the FDA approval process has resulted in low-profit margin, low-patient-volume and rare-disease drugs not even being developed or brought to market.

The FDA also regulates development and release of medical devices, such as joint prostheses, pacemakers and artificial heart valves. The agency uses the same bureaucratic approach to medical device research as it takes with drug development. Clinical trials in Europe, for example, take much less time than in the U.S. and consequently devices and drugs can help needy patients much more quickly.

7.
MEDICARE

The establishment of Medicare was discussed above, but since it is the largest socialized health care program in the world, it bears further examination to see how far we've progressed with it. As mentioned, at Medicare's outset in 1965 at least 60 percent of all seniors already had some form of health insurance. Also, low income seniors were provided with health insurance on a voluntary basis through the Kerr-Mills law of 1960. These facts raise the question of why a new program was needed, whether Medicare was simply pandering to the senior vote, and whether Medicare was being used as the first step to complete socialization of health care in the U.S.

From the start, the cost of the Medicare program was grossly underestimated. The Health, Education, and Welfare Department told Congress in 1965 that the funding would require much less than 1 percent of payroll taxes. By the late 1980s, however, this was increased to 1.6 percent. In dollar amounts, spending on Medicare was $4.6 billion in 1967 but had increased to $7.9 billion by 1971. This represented a 22 percent increase in cost-adjusted dollars, whereas enrollment had increased only six percent.

In 2009, 47 million seniors received their health insurance from Medicare at a cost of $500 billion. At the current rate of growth, it is estimated that Medicare costs will almost double in ten years to $940 billion in 2019.

The current Medicare payroll tax is at 2.9 percent and will increase to 3.8 percent for high wage earners after PPACA takes effect in 2014. If all Medicare deficits were to be covered, the payroll tax should have been raised to 18 percent in 2004, and to provide a break even cash flow, each worker should have paid 20 percent in 2008. A payroll tax increase of this magnitude is not politically or economically possible, especially when stacked on top of worker income taxes.

Figure 3
Projected vs. Actual Medicare Tax Burden:
Combined Employee/Employer Maximum Tax Rate
for Financing Medicare Part A

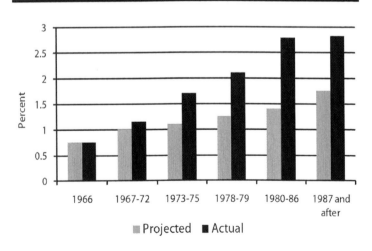

The taxable wage basis initially was $6,600. By 1993, Congress had increased the wage basis to $135,000 and the following year this cap was eliminated completely, so that all wages were taxable in an attempt to cover skyrocketing Medicare expenses.

Figure 4
General Revenue Transfers to Medicare as a Share of Federal Income Tax Revenue

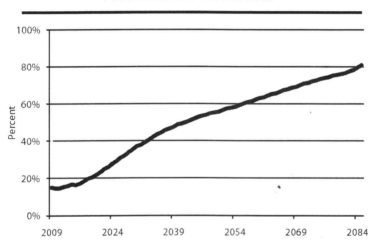

Like Social Security, Medicare was set up as a pay-as-you-go system, where benefits are funded by current taxes, but the first wave of recipients had contributed nothing in payroll tax to the program. And, with the decreasing number of workers in future generations, and with the massive number of baby boomers approaching retirement, this pay-as-you-go system is a catastrophe waiting to happen.

Likewise, the Johnson administration's belief that increasing the number of hospitals and doctors would increase competition and bring costs down also proved to be false logic. Unfortunately, their economic model broke down because they evidently forgot that seniors were not spending their own money for the health care they were receiving. So, no surprise, demand for free health care went up and supply was increased as access was made easier. Clearly, two wrongs did not make a right. For example, the number of operations on seniors increased two and a half times in the first ten years of Medicare, in spite of a fairly constant enrollment (Pearman and Starr 1988, p.23).

As with so many bureaucratic government programs, Medicare is associated with a significant amount of waste. It is estimated that fraud, abuse, and waste together cost almost $12 billion per year (U.S. Dept. of Health and Human Services report, 2001). Approximately 20 percent of Medicare spending provides no benefit in lives saved or in improved quality of life for our senior citizens.

From the outset of Medicare, one glaring deficiency has persisted. This is the fact that the program provides no catastrophic coverage. It provides first-dollar health care maintenance, but after a certain point the program stops paying. In 2001 dollars, Medicare paid $192 per day for the first 60 days of hospitalization, $198 for days 61-90, and $396 for days 91-150.

After 150 days, the senior is required to pay 100 percent out of pocket. Again, this structure is pretty much the opposite of true indemnity insurance.

Tragically, today's seniors are paying almost as much out of pocket for health care through their Medicare co-pay as they were for private insurance prior to the passage of the Medicare bill. It is projected that seniors will be paying approximately 30 percent of their income for Medicare coverage by 2025 (Moon, 1999).

Figure 5
Acute Health Spending by the Elderly
(Percentage of Income)

What about bang for the buck? From the outset, Medicare reimbursed states differently based on health care expenses regionally. It is very clear now, after forty years, that seniors in the higher-reimbursed states have no better longevity or quality of life. Life expectancy was already on the rise before 1965 and showed no dramatic increase after the passage of Medicare (Bureau of the Census, 1975).

Since the late 1980s, Congress has been gradually decreasing hospital and physician reimbursements. Just like any other government wage-and-price control policy, supply is reduced, and seniors' access to health care is now being restricted. In many communities throughout the nation, seniors are finding decreasing access to primary care because doctors can't cover their overhead with Medicare's reimbursements. Clearly this restricts seniors' health care choices. It should also be noted that Medicare law requires that if a physician accepts payment for a senior's health care from a source other than Medicare, that doctor can then not accept any Medicare patients for two years. Because the private insurance market for seniors has essentially been eliminated in the U.S., even the wealthier elderly have no other option other than to participate in Medicare. Doctors cannot accept cash or private insurance and still serve Medicare patients.

It is Medicare Part B that reimburses physicians. Not surprisingly, Congress had no budget schedule for Part B. It was originally set up so that seniors would pay part and the federal government would match that to cover doctors' fees. In 1967 the total cost of Part B was $2 billion, but by 2000, the total expense was $90 billion. Taxpayers were funding 75 percent of that $90 billion instead of the originally proposed 50 percent match.

Through the years the federal government has placed many additional restrictions and regulatory burdens on the Medicare program. One of the most recent and wide sweeping is the Health Insurance Portability and Accountability Act of 1996 (HIPAA). Although originally intended to create an electronic national health information system, by 2001 HIPAA had morphed into an unenforceable, bureaucratic patient-confidentiality nightmare for health care providers. It gives the government the authority to determine who can see a patient's private records even without that person's consent, although providers may not freely discuss a patient's case. This is but one example of the government manipulating the practice of medicine once it is paying for the care. As is true everywhere, whoever pays the bill runs the show.

Not only is Medicare nearly bankrupt now, but its future is actually much more dismal. With a decreasing labor force and an increasing number of seniors over the age of sixty-five, the Medicare pay-as-you-go system is on a collision course for disaster. Most young people in their twenties and thirties do not believe the program will be there for them when they reach age sixty-five.

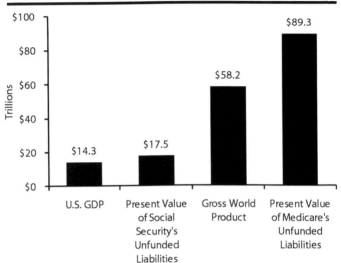

Figure 6
Medicare's Unfunded Liabilities Compared
with Other Measures, 2009

If Medicare is to continue in its present form, one or more of three things must happen: benefits will need to be decreased, payroll taxes will need to be increased, or seniors will need to pay more out of pocket. A fourth option, of course, would be to use the general tax fund to cover more of Medicare deficits. From an economic standpoint, none of these things would predictably rein in the costs or decrease the demand for health care on the part of Medicare beneficiaries.

It is somewhat unbelievable that people are calling for complete socialization of health care in the U.S. when Medicare, a socialized-medicine program itself, has been in such a dismal financial condition since its inception. By the mid-twentieth-first century, Medicare expenditures will dwarf the cost of Social Security.

PPACA dramatically cuts over $500 billion from the Medicare program over the first ten years. Medicare clearly needs reform, but the new legislation reduces doctor and hospital reimbursement by over $400 billion and essentially eliminates Medicare Part C, or Medicare Advantage.

Although these planned doctor and hospital cuts may not happen ultimately, it is obvious that supporters of PPACA want to fund the new entitlement programs by reducing doctor payments in Medicare. This will make access to health care for seniors all the more difficult.

8.
MEDICAID

The Medicaid program, which was part of the Medicare bill of 1965, provided both federal and state funding for health care for the poor and disabled.

There are currently four groups of people receiving assistance through the Medicaid program. These are the poor, the disabled, mothers and children, and those individuals needing long-term care. Although mothers and children make up most of the beneficiaries, long-term care accounts for 70 percent of Medicaid dollars spent.

Medicaid expenditures are the fastest-growing budget item for virtually all states, even though the federal government supplies, on average, 57 percent of all Medicaid dollars spent. State reimbursement by the federal government is based on the wealth of the state, with poorer states receiving a higher percentage match of federal money than wealthier ones.

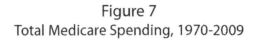

Figure 7
Total Medicare Spending, 1970-2009

Physician participation is voluntary, and doctor reimbursement from Medicaid has always been lower than that of any other insurance carrier, including Medicare. Consequently, an increasing number of physicians are withdrawing from the program, thus decreasing beneficiaries' access to health care by limiting their physician choices.

The cost of Medicaid was $1 billion its first year, exploding to $430 billion by 2009. At the present rate of growth, the cost will be $900 billion by 2019 (over ten years), and by the year 2030, it is estimated that nursing home expenditures alone will equal the size of the entire Social Security program today.

Medicaid has resulted in a number of harmful conse-quences. First, it discourages work and job improvement for low-paid employees, since with increasing income workers lose their Medicaid benefits. It also encourages low-wage paying employers to not offer health benefits. They assume, or hope, taxpayers will provide those benefits. Medicaid also discourages private insurance companies from offering nursing-home poli-cies, and this market shrinks more every year. Lastly, Medicaid discourages charity care and philanthropic work in the health care sector – if the government is already funding health care, donors are more likely to contribute money to other causes.

State lawmakers unfortunately are caught in a vicious cycle where the more they spend on Medicaid, the more money they receive from the federal government. In other words, if a state spends one dollar on education, it receives one dollar's worth of education. However, if a state spends one dollar on Medicaid benefits, it gets two dollars of health care, because of matching funds from the federal government. It is therefore no surprise that Medicaid is the largest, and fastest growing, budget item for almost all states in the country.

Many states are now looking for ways to extract themselves from federal control of Medicaid. States are finding the open-ended entitlement is one of the main drivers of chronic budget deficits. The states are asking for block-grants from the federal government so individual states can then establish their own health care program for their poor residents.

PPACA will add sixteen to twenty-three million more people to Medicaid. Although these people will have health "insurance," they will find their actual access to health care is very limited.

9.
COSTS

Total health care costs in the United States account for almost 18 percent of our gross domestic product (GDP). It is true that this is a higher percentage than any other country, but much of this difference is because of our higher GDP. The richer the country, the more health care it can afford.

Third-party payers, in other words someone other than the patient, pay for 88 percent of health care in the United States. The government, the largest third-party payer, pays for 50 percent of all health care in our country, much of it through Medicare and Medicaid.

In 2009, the federal government spent $500 billion on Medicare. It is estimated this number will increase to $940 billion within ten years (2019). Medicaid spending by both federal and state governments totaled $430 billion in 2009 and even without PPACA, Medicaid costs are projected to reach $900 billion in 2019. If no changes are made, by 2030, the two programs alone will account for 11 percent of our GDP.

Although Medicare is essentially a pay-as-you-go system, a lump sum of over $100 trillion would need to be deposited today in an interest-bearing account to cover future promises for all those people currently enrolled or who have contributed to Medicare. This amount is more than double the combined GDPs of all countries and is more than seven times higher than the GDP of the United States. Obviously, sustaining Medicare is a huge problem.

For the past sixteen years, health care costs for employers and employees have risen faster than both inflation and workers' earnings. Cost increases have routinely exceeded 10 percent per year, which has the effect of decreasing wages by 2.3 percent and, unfortunately, eliminating certain lower-paying jobs.

The individual private health insurance market is no better off, with rates increasing much faster than both inflation and the cost of living. This has resulted in more people being priced out of the private health insurance market and more patients seeking routine care in an expensive emergency department setting.

It is estimated that over 20 percent of men and over 30 percent of women stay at their existing jobs because of fear of losing their health benefits (Adams, 2004).

Many people believe a socialized health care system would decrease administrative costs and thereby decrease overall health care costs. Research suggests, however, that more bureaucracy would add to administrative expenses. Once all hidden costs are considered, Canada's socialized medicine program has an overhead of almost 45 percent (Danzon, 1992). By comparison, most private plans in the U.S. have an overhead of less than 10 percent, clearly less than the cost of administering Medicare and Medicaid.

It also seems logical that more preventive medicine would lower health care costs. For certain diseases and certain patients this may be true, but, unfortunately, for the overall health care bill, there is no decrease in cost. Early detection of disease can save money, but the cost of screening every person for every disease is prohibitive.

By some estimates, we could spend our entire GDP today if every test and procedure were done for every person in the U.S. Obviously, this is ridiculous, but the corollary is that someone has to decide which patients receive what tests. Should it be the patient and doctor, or should it be the bureaucrats?

One final huge contributor to cost in the U.S. is our legal system. It is estimated that up to 20 percent of our health care spending is a direct result of the litigious nature of our justice system. (For more about the costs of health care tied to our legal system, see Chapter 15).

10.
OTHER COUNTRIES

We have long heard the argument that the United States is the only industrialized country without socialized medicine. The logic is that if everyone else has it, socialized, single-payer health care must be the best solution to our current crisis. Let's look at those other countries and see whether they actually do function well and if they would be applicable to our society (Tanner, 2008).

GERMANY

Germany was the first country to institute a form of socialized health care, starting in 1883. Today German health care consumes 11 percent of GDP. Payroll taxes to finance the program are at 13 percent of gross wages, with payment split between employer and employee. These matching funds go to 1,400 nonprofit insurance companies to which everyone must belong. The unemployed are enrolled and paid for by the government.

Although the 1,400 insurance funds set their own fees for hospital and doctor reimbursement, those prices and wages are heavily regulated by the federal government.

Patients pay a small fee for drugs and hospital stays.

The latest national survey reveals that 20 percent of Germans experienced waiting times of more than twelve weeks for specialist or surgical care. Almost 55 percent of Germans think their system needs reform, while only 35 percent give their health care high marks (www.dw-world.de/2007).

In 2003, the Ministry of Health reported the German health care system suffered from a "lack of competition, superfluous, inappropriate or insufficient care, decreasing revenue, and an aging population." Their health care deficit at that time was three billion euros. Plans for correction include increasing patient co-payments, increasing competition, and decreasing unemployment.

GREAT BRITAIN

Great Britain established the first comprehensive health care system (the NHC) in the free world in 1948. This program is essentially a cradle-to-grave entitlement for every citizen. The country gives open access to primary care, although the general practitioner may not be of the patient's choosing. With over one million employees, the NHC is one of the world's largest employers.

There are very modest drug co-pays and basically no hospital or physician charges. The NHC is financed largely through the general tax, plus a small percent from payroll taxes.

About 10 percent of the population has private insurance, and many physicians combine NHC work with their private practice.

The current wait to enter the hospital for a number of procedures is up to one year, and, through the 1990s, over one million British patients were on government lists waiting for care. Inefficiencies are rampant, and chronic shortages, with resulting rationing, are commonplace.

JAPAN

Japan socialized its health delivery system in 1961, when the country required everyone to join a health insurance plan directed by the government. The entire system is essentially a pay-as-you-go plan. Retirees, self-employed, and unemployed are covered by the National Health Insurance Plan (NHIP), and workers are enrolled in one of the various employee plans. The NHIP is funded by the government and the employee plans are funded equally by employers and workers. Monthly premiums differ based on salary.

Since 1995, when extrapolation of spending trends revealed that by year 2025 Japan would be consuming 50 percent of its GDP for medical care, the Japanese system has undergone gradual reform (www.sq.emb-japan.go.jp/JapanAccess/health.htm, 2007). Japan is experiencing an increasing senior population and a decreasing birth rate, making for an unsustainable health delivery system.

Seniors now must pay an increased fixed premium and worker co-pays have gone from 10 percent to 20 percent. Likewise, physician reimbursement has been adjusted downward and continues to be re-evaluated. In spite of these changes, most reports indicate the current Japanese medical insurance system is on the verge of bankruptcy.

CANADA

A change to a Canadian-type health care system is frequently discussed in the United States. Canada socialized its medical program in 1971. Every citizen is covered with no co-payment for primary care and essentially free choice of physicians.

The system is financed with 50 percent federal money and 50 percent provincial taxpayer funds, although the poorer provinces pay less. Dollars come from both income and sales tax, with up to 20 percent of the budget provided by payroll deductions. The income tax rate is almost 50 percent in Canada.

Supplemental insurance, often provided by employers, is available to pay for certain procedures not covered by the national plan. Seniors over the age of sixty-four, the unemployed, and the poor pay no premiums and have no out-of-pocket expenses for health care.

Most hospitals are private, and an insurance program in each province reimburses its hospitals on the basis of cost.

Acceptable costs are determined by a governmental rate-setting committee in each province. Physicians are fee-for-service, but the provincial medical association sets their fees for all services.

Although primary care is generally available, specialty care and diagnostic procedures are in short supply because of lack of funding. Long waiting lists are commonplace. Likewise, there has been a significant brain drain of Canadian physicians, as they come to the U.S. because of their frustration with the system and poor reimbursement.

Just recently a few provinces, experiencing high cost overruns, have experimented with a formal second tier of private insurance and reimbursement. It is too early to accurately determine the impact of this liberalization. For years, however, the United States has served as Canada's medical safety valve, an alternative source of health care for Canadians unwilling to wait for tests or procedures in their own country.

SWITZERLAND

Switzerland uses a model of government "managed competition" with an individual mandate to purchase health insurance. It is not employer-based and relies on "private" insurers that must honor guaranteed issue (i.e. must sell to anyone regardless of pre-existing health conditions) and community rating (all people except for smokers are in the same risk pool).

Individuals in Switzerland pay approximately 30 percent of their health care expenses out-of-pocket and the government subsidizes nearly one third of all Swiss citizens.

Insurance companies set provider prices in a cartel fashion and compete on policy price and benefits. Basic benefits packages are determined by the government. Because of special interests, the political influence of the government is constantly expanding the basic benefit package.

Because employers are not involved, the Swiss are exposed to the full cost of their health care. This has led to a greater degree of consumerism in health care than in other countries. Yet because the list of government mandated benefits in any insurance plan continues to grow, the Swiss are paying more and finding fewer options for health insurance.

RATIONING

One last, very important point is that the demand for health care far outstrips the money budgeted for it in all of these countries. The results of this demand/supply mismatch are chronic shortages followed by rationing of health care. The rationing can take many forms - from long waits, to not providing the elderly with certain procedures, to allowing individuals with political influence to have priority.

The actual winners in a bureaucratic rationing system are the affluent, the healthy, the young, white males, and the politically powerful. The losers are everyone else.

11.
QUALITY OF CARE

There is a general sense that we are not getting our money's worth for all the health spending in this country. The inference is that other countries spend less and get better care. What is the reality?

Let's start with infant mortality. The United States would appear to have a higher infant mortality rate than most other industrialized nations, based on data from the Organization for Economic Cooperation and Development (OECD report, 2004). The data from the U.S., however, includes all live births, whereas most other countries do not automatically include premature and low-birth-weight babies. This fact, coupled with the heterogeneity of the U.S. population, can explain virtually all of the infant mortality difference.

Life expectancy is another factor used when comparing health spending by country; however, there is absolutely no correlation between the two among industrialized nations. The argument that we should live longer because we spend more money does not hold up to any inter-country comparison.

Plus, the U.S. has a higher rate of homicides and major trauma than other western countries. Murder and car accidents reflect socio-economic problems, but do not have anything to do with a country's health care delivery system.

Quality of life is another issue and, because of its subjective nature, it has never been studied in a nation-by-nation comparison. It makes sense, though, that most people in the industrialized world are comfortable with their lifestyles and would believe their quality of life to be good.

There is a strong correlation between a country's GDP and the amount of health care it uses. It is estimated that up to 90 percent of the difference between health care spending in the U.S. and other countries is because of our higher GDP (Reinhardt and Hussey, 2004). The richer the country, the more it spends on health care.

Medical errors are another factor to look at when comparing the quality of our health care system with those of other industrialized nations. Does our system lead to more medical errors than these countries' systems? The most recent reports indicate that between 46,000 and 98,000 deaths per year in the U.S. are caused by errors. A careful review of these cases by a physician panel, however, concluded that many of these deaths occurred at the end of life or in critically ill patients, where death was the most likely outcome regardless of the care the patient received (Hayward and Hofer, 2001).

A comparative study done in Canada, the poster child for a single -payer system, found 9,250 to 23,750 deaths per year that met the "medical error" criteria (Canada Institute for Health Information report, 2004). If these numbers were adjusted for the larger U.S. population, they would be 83,000 to 214,000. So actually, it appears our "broken" system results in fewer deaths due to medical errors than the Canadian single-payer system.

It is often said that our health care system ranks 37th in the world. This ranking is from a study done in the late 1990s by the World Health Organization (CATO Briefing Paper, 2008). The study was designed to look at five fundamental health delivery criteria, in which three of the five were based on whether a country has a government-run, single payer type system. The U.S. has a hybrid system composed of both private and government health care. Consequently, the United States was at a disadvantage in 60 percent of the measures used in the study. France was ranked number one and the U.S. was ranked behind Greece, Colombia and Morocco, for example. It is laughable to think anyone in the U.S. would want to travel to Morocco for their health care.

We do know that for all we spend, compared to other countries, our technology is better and more prevalent, waiting times for tests and procedures are shorter, and in general patients are very satisfied with the quality of the care they receive.

12.
FIRST-DOLLAR COVERAGE AND THIRD-PARTY PAYMENT

Costs for health care in the United States have exploded in the past sixty years. In inflation-adjusted dollars, the average spent per person was $82 in 1950, $183 in 1986, and over $5,000 today. Third parties, either employers or the government, pay for 88 percent of health care today in our country. The government alone finances nearly half of all our health spending.

Figure 8
Real Health Care Expenditures and 3rd-Party Payments

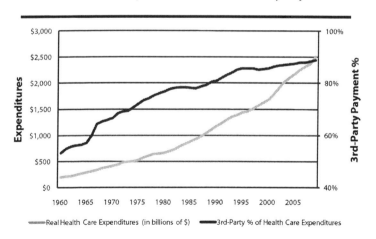

The fact that a third party pays for health care hides the actual costs from both the patient (the consumer) and the doctor (the provider). There realistically is no incentive for the patient or doctor to limit or restrict the amount of health care used or offered, because from their point of view, someone else will pay the bill.

Figure 9
Shifting Modes of Financing Health Care, 1965-2001

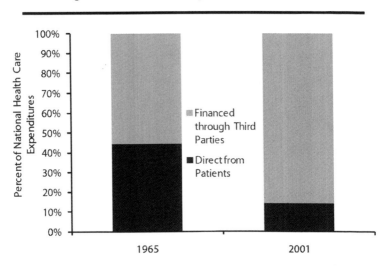

The economic result of cost being disconnected from demand is high rates of overutilization. In a recent study, families with unlimited health care, compared to families with a high-deductible insurance policy of several thousand dollars, used 43 percent more care, with no difference in health outcomes (Newhouse, 1996, p. 338-339).

As an analogy, let's say 88 percent of the car owners in the U.S. could choose any auto they wanted and someone else would pay for the vehicle and all its upkeep. If you are among the 88 percent, why drive a Chevy when you could drive a Lexus? Why own a Miata when you could drive a Corvette? And why conserve gas when someone else is paying for it? Why maintain your car when you know someone else will buy you a new one next year?

This car scenario is laughable, but unfortunately, it is the exact situation we have in health care in the United States. The supply and demand mismatch would only get worse with a single-payer, socialized system.

But, you say, the government would limit health care expenses and costs, so everyone couldn't drive the car of their choice - to mix analogies. Fair enough, but then the government would decide who receives health care and how much. The government would decide who drives what car based on some bureaucratic formula. In other words, rationing would, by necessity, take place with paternalistic bureaucrats making health decisions for each of us.

One of the most common arguments made against a free market in health care, versus a socialized system, is the lack of patient education in making informed decisions. When people spend their own money, however, they are much more likely to seek and obtain the information they need to make informed, appropriate decisions. What is lacking today is a mechanism for people to obtain that knowledge. In this age of information and advertising, there is no reason patients cannot become informed consumers of health care, just as car buyers research different makes and models of cars when deciding what vehicle best suits their driving needs. In a free market, such things as consumer reports, comparison shopping and word-of-mouth provide education for smart shoppers. The same principle applies to medicine. Certainly in this computer and internet age, consumers have access, at their fingertips, to a robust amount of health care information.

What about the emergency nature of medicine? How does a person make an informed choice in the middle of a heart attack or stroke or major accident? It turns out that almost 85 percent of health care in the United States is routine and only about 15 percent is of an emergent nature (Ricardo-Campbell, 1982, p.93). For most of the medical care needed and received, the patient has time to become a knowledgeable consumer. In a free and open insurance market, competitive policies for emergency care would be available to individuals before their emergencies. Likewise, community standards for emergency care could be established, just as we have with fire fighting and 911 services.

What is the impact of third-party payers on patient and doctor interaction? In the days before Medicare and Medicaid and employers paying for workers' health care, people dealt with their hospitals and doctors in a more or less free-market manner. Patients were not denied treatment if they did not pay, but a general understanding existed that non-indigent people were responsible for the costs of their own medical care. Over the past sixty years, we have gradually moved away from this responsibility, with devastating consequences.

The most fundamental problem now is that patients, health care providers and even hospitals have no idea of the true costs of specific medical treatments, as discussed above. Patients are aware that their insurance premiums or their Medicare co-pays are going up, and taxpayers understand that Medicare and Medicaid costs are rising. Yet in spite of a general sense that medical results are improving, there is no specific correlation in the public's mind between better value and rising health care costs.

In a truly free market, the consumer (or patient) could see and experience the effects of competition and improving technology. One has to look no further than the automobile or cellular-phone industry to see examples of how technology is improving the product and at the same time bringing costs down.

Competition has not occurred in the health field, and it is easy to understand why. In the present medical environment, there is virtually no mechanism for price comparisons and no way to obtain cost-versus-outcome relationships. With someone else paying for a patient's health care, there is absolutely no incentive for the patient to look for less expensive alternatives, no incentive for physicians to inform patients of various treatment costs (even if they knew those costs), and no mechanism for hospitals to ethically and legally advertise their rates and costs.

The motivator for cost awareness in health care would be eliminating third-party payers and allowing patients to provide and control their own health care dollars. This is really the only economic model that allows patients (the most interested parties) to pay for their medical decisions with their own money. The resulting enormous health care consumer movement, made up of patients, would drive cost efficiency in the medical arena. The lack of cost information today is a direct result of a relatively disinterested party (an employer or the government) paying for medical care of a very interested person (the patient).

Of course, as health care costs have skyrocketed, the payers are definitely becoming more interested in these escalating expenses, though not in the quality of care. We are rapidly reaching the tipping point where employers and state governments are, unfortunately, looking to the federal government for a solution. The only alternative in many payers' minds today is a socialized, government-controlled, single-payer system. This, sadly, does not take into consideration the best interests and desires of health care users. Just as most people in this country control the dollars they spend on food, clothing and shelter, so too should they have the genuine ability to control their health care dollars. The only mechanism to allow this control is the elimination of third-party payment and the establishment of an economic structure to provide true individual health care insurance, not health maintenance.

13.
HEALTH CARE INSURANCE TODAY

Merriam Webster's Collegiate Dictionary, Eleventh Edition, defines insurance as "coverage by contract whereby one party undertakes to indemnify or guarantee another against loss by a specified contingency or peril." This is the accepted definition when we think of car or home insurance, but clearly this is not what "health insurance" has come to mean.

Health insurance is essentially pre-paid health maintenance. We now expect that our health insurance will pay for not only major or emergent problems, but that it will also cover routine care such as doctor visits, prescription drugs, and even eye glasses in some cases.

We do not expect our car or home insurance to cover routine maintenance such as brake repair or plumbing repair, but we do buy insurance to cover such things as major collisions and home fires.

The fact that someone else is paying for this health care maintenance only makes overutilization predictable and inevitable. Who wouldn't want someone else to pay for their car maintenance or their routine home repair?

This third party payer mentality for both routine and emergent care has created an economic situation that logically can't sustain itself, because the cost is driven by the unlimited demand. It is no wonder our health care as a percentage of gross domestic product is growing so rapidly.

14.
UNINSURED

Much of the demand for change in our health delivery system is based on the rising number of people without insurance. We have already explored the misnomer of health "insurance," which is actually health "maintenance," so let's move on to the uninsured group. In 2010, there were approximately fifty million people who did not have health insurance for at least one day that year.

As it turns out, only about 15 percent of people without insurance remain uninsured for more than two years. The majority of these individuals are either changing jobs or are just entering the job market. Others are caught up in an insurance waiting period or are students with part-time jobs (Henderson, 2002). Also, nearly 30 percent of the uninsured already qualify for an existing plan, such as Medicaid, but are unaware of the program or have decided not to sign up for it (Congressional Budget Office, 2003).

Almost 50 percent of the uninsured are 18 to 34 years old. These people are young and healthy. They are either still in school or are just starting out in the work force, typically in a low-paying job. Health insurance is not a priority for them and not buying insurance is often a rational economic decision. Many young adults have been priced out of the individual insurance market by state mandates imposed on private insurance. The irony here, of course, is that these people would have access to insurance if politicians cut back on regulations and allowed a free market in health coverage.

There is also the issue of people not having insurance even when they can afford it - the so called "free riders" on the system. Although a lot has been written about this group, interestingly enough, they account for less than 3 percent of all health care spending in the United States, according to an editorial in *The Wall Street Journal* on May 2, 2006. Consequently, it makes no sense to use this group as a reason for imposing mandatory insurance or a single payer system on everyone.

Finally, the most important people in this debate are the chronically uninsured – those who year after year go without health insurance. This group contains approximately ten million people, which is not a small number. Yet, ten million is less than 3 percent of the U.S. population and is a disingenuous reason for a total government takeover of our health care system.

15.
MEDICAL MALPRACTICE

It is estimated that up to 20 percent of all health spending in the United States is the result of our legal system. This 20 percent figure includes malpractice premiums, actual court and attorney fees, settlements and judgments, and defensive medical practices. The legal costs and the litigious nature of this country in general must be factored into any comparison of our health care system with other countries' systems.

It should be noted that in many cases providers are sued for bad outcomes and not for malpractice. When dealing with the human body, poor results can often occur in unexpected ways without a negligent cause.

Physicians in the U.S. are seeing dramatically escalating costs of malpractice premiums, especially in high risk specialties. Some communities and patient groups are already experiencing physician shortages in high-risk fields like obstetrics, neurosurgery, and trauma care.

Congress has not dealt with this issue and probably rightfully so, since there is no provision for it in the Constitution. Since it therefore is a state issue, let's look at the states that have enacted meaningful medical liability reform.

First of all, those states have experienced either no physician shortage or have seen an improvement in an existing shortage. Physicians choose to locate in states with a stable overhead environment, rather than worry from year to year about rising malpractice insurance premiums.

Secondly, these states do not deny injured patients their day in court. They place no cap on economic damages and maintenance fees, but do place significant caps on pain and suffering awards. These caps on non-economic damages have been the most effective method of controlling runaway jury awards that in turn lead to skyrocketing malpractice premiums. These states also placed caps on the amount lawyers can collect in these cases, so that more of the judgment money goes to the patient.

Likewise, many states passed joint and several liability reform and made other income sources for the plaintiff discoverable (Gingrich and Gill, 2006). These reforms allow juries to assign blame accurately, so one party, the doctor, does not bear full responsibility when several people are at fault.

Pre-trial screening and arbitration panels show potential for allowing patients access to the legal system while holding down the cost of malpractice awards. States are also exploring the qualifications of expert witnesses and considering statute-of-limitations on medical malpractices cases (McQuillan and Abramyan, 2010).

Other proposals for medical liability reform include a loser-pay system to discourage frivolous lawsuits and a fund outside the legal system that would pay injured patients, like a workers' compensation program.

16.
HEALTH CARE AS A RIGHT

For the past century the belief that health care is a right has been growing in this country. It is now widely accepted that every member of our society has some type of privilege, or right, to receive medical treatment. Although the Declaration of Independence mentions "life," "liberty" and "the pursuit of happiness," it never addresses the government's role in health care.

If we accept health care as a right, then there are a few problems we must address.

For starters, how much medical care should each person receive? In other words, should every person get all screening tests, all procedures, all medicines, and unlimited treatment? To do that today would consume 100 percent of our gross domestic product.

So if each person should not receive unlimited care, who decides how much care a person receives and who those people should be? This, of course, is problem number two. Do we leave the decisions to the patients and the medical community or to government bureaucrats? If we choose the bureaucracy, than we will have to accept the inefficiencies, the political power struggles, and the lack of personal involvement that we see in our present government programs.

Problem number three is who pays and how much is paid? Do we use a payroll tax, a general income tax, a national sales tax, or some other creative tax program? Should there be a co-payment or unlimited care? Remember, realistically, we can't afford total care for everyone, so should our politicians decide how much health care each of us needs?

A final problem is the incentive structure for patients and health care workers. From an economic standpoint, if something is free, utilization will increase. This is a virtual law of nature or, at least, of economics. There would be no incentive to not use as much health care as possible.

The incentive for nurses, medical technicians and physicians works in the opposite direction. Who would be willing to spend eight to twelve years after college to train as doctors only to have their income controlled by bureaucrats and be paid considerably less than expected for their level of education and responsibility? Likewise, would future nurses and technicians be as willing to enter the profession knowing they had no choice but to be paid as government employees?

It would seem what health-care-as-a-right advocates really mean is they believe **access** to health care is a right, just as people believe they should have access to food and shelter. None of us thinks we can fill our cart at the grocery store and walk out without paying. No one believes all housing should be free. We do believe government exists to provide a free market in food and shelter, however, so we can find competitive food stores and housing.

Similarly, the government should provide a platform for the free market delivery of health care. The tragedy is we do not have a truly free market in medical care in this country. Medicine today is one of the most heavily regulated industries in the U.S., and to believe the current system is a free market is totally erroneous.

Almost from the birth of the nation, the government has been involved in health care delivery, regulation, and licensure. Over half of the people in the U.S. are now covered by government-sponsored, taxpayer-funded health plans. The bureaucrats dictate private insurance rates and coverage mandates. Yet even with the government as heavily involved as it is, health care costs are escalating far beyond the cost of living.

The new PPACA health care law essentially gives government complete control of our health care system. Everyone will be forced to purchase health insurance; Medicaid will be widely expanded; benefits and prices for private insurance in the exchanges will be set by bureaucrats; taxpayer subsidies for insurance will be available not only for the poor, but also the middle class; and finally, the government will establish agencies that determine "best practices," determining who gets how much and what kind of health care.

There is no reason to believe that expanded involvement or total control of our health care by the government will result in less cost and improved quality. Unless we have government rationing, costs can only be controlled by supply and demand in a competitive free market. And, there is no reason to believe rationing will lead to better quality health care. Consumerism in health care would improve quality, just as we have seen in other economic areas such as computers, cellular phones and automobiles.

17.
THE DOCTOR SHORTAGE

Ever since the Flexner Report was published in the early twentieth century, the government has controlled physician education and supply in the U.S. Medical school licensure is determined by the federal government and doctor licenses are issued by state governments.

Part of the Medicare law in 1965 provided extra funding for institutions that train medical students, interns and residents. Medicare funding now accounts for two thirds of the cost of training a doctor. Consequently, the physician supply in the U.S. has been largely determined by the level of federal funding. Congress set a limit in 1996 on the number of new doctors Medicare would finance. Recently, the government has proposed an additional $60 billion cut in Medicare for doctor training through 2020.

The new federal health care reform law will give thirty-two million more people in the U.S. health insurance. Last year, forty-six million seniors received health care through the Medicare program and with the aging of the baby boomer population

Medicare is expected to cover seventy-two million people by 2020. So at the same time the government is reducing the number of doctors, the central planners in Washington, D.C., are adding almost sixty million new patients to our health care system.

The U.S. now trains approximately 16,000 new doctors each year. To keep up with the sixty million additionally insured patients, the country would need to train almost 24,000 physicians every year. With the cuts in Medicare funding, the number of doctors trained will actually fall to less than today's 16,000 per year. Also, surveys reveal that almost one third of practicing physicians today (about 250,000) are over the age of 55 and plan to retire by 2020 (Pardes, 2011). This, of course, will simply compound the impending doctor shortage in our country.

One last point, unfortunately, is that with more government control, a career in medicine will look much less attractive to bright high school and college students. Why spend four years in medical school and three to seven additional years in internship and residency training so one can end up working for the government? In addition, bureaucrats will determine "best practices" (in other words, who gets care and what kind of care they receive), they will set provider reimbursement levels, and they will determine how many primary care and specialists should be trained. Our best students will find many other career choices more attractive than health care.

18.
SOLUTIONS

The economic system that made our country prosper and grow is the free market. From affordable transportation, to affordable housing, to affordable food, our system of relatively free interaction between buyer and seller has allowed technology to blossom and has provided us with a standard of living unparalleled in world history. There is nothing unique about health care delivery, except for historical precedence, that would not allow the same free market system to flourish in this country.

Unfortunately, and predictably, our current hybrid system of part socialized medicine coupled with a heavily regulated "free" market is not sustainable. A completely socialized, government-run single-payer system limits patient choice, causes rationing, and restricts technological advancement. It is based on bureaucratic decision-making for patients and health care deliverers; it is inefficient, and it results in chronic underfunding in spite of high taxation.

Those who advocate a socialized, single-payer system as a solution to our health care problems must first explain why the government bureaucracy would be more efficient than the free market, why it would cost less, and why health care rationing is good for patients.

Innovation occurs in the free market. New technologies and procedures are discovered and developed in an arena without the stifling processes of government bureaucracies. Government central planning and "pilot" programs do not result in innovative solutions for patients. There are thousands of undiscovered solutions to our health care problems, but only in a free market will these discoveries be allowed to flourish and grow into practical treatments that relieve human suffering.

At present, there are basically five solutions to our current health care problem, and they are described below. Individually, each would help relieve our problem. Together, they provide a complete answer. It will take political courage to reach the endpoint, however. And political courage is really about leadership and about explaining to people what will work - not necessarily promising them something for nothing in order to get re-elected.

1) CHANGE THE TAX CODE

First of all, we must change the federal tax code and allow individuals to deduct their health expenses just as businesses and privately insured self-employed individuals do. This would give employees the freedom to purchase their own insurance and would allow employers to decrease their overhead and, potentially, offer higher wages. It would provide larger insurance pools of many individuals from many companies, rather than a single, company-based pool. It would potentially give employees a greater choice in the type and amount of insurance coverage.

Since World War II, there has been a movement in the U.S. toward employer-provided health care, and employees have come to expect it. Yet the individual tax savings and greater freedom of choice would more than make up for the current employer-provided system. The real question is why should a business be able to deduct health benefits for its employees, but the workers themselves can't? It makes no sense.

Individual insurance coverage, not tied to a certain employer, would also allow for portability of health care coverage. Workers could move from one job to another, from state to state if necessary, and retain their own health insurance.

Another related question is why should an employer provide health care benefits in the first place? Why not simply adjust wages up and allow employees to purchase their own individual plans? Except for retirement plans, there are very few other benefits provided by employers.

Critics say we need a healthy work force and therefore it is in an employer's best interest to provide health insurance. But we also need a well-fed, clothed and sheltered work force. Employers are not involved in these activities. There is no reason, except for the accident of history, to treat health care for employees differently than these other necessities of life.

It will take a change in mind-set across the country to eliminate the notion that employers should provide employee health benefits.

2) ELIMINATE STATE MANDATES

Mandates set by state legislatures now restrict patient choice in the purchase of individual health insurance. Instead of offering a buffet of programs, mandates require all individual plans to provide the same benefits. Why should a twenty-five-year-old, single man be required to pay for obstetrical coverage? Why should anyone be forced to pay for chiropractic or mental health coverage if they don't want it?

Supporters of mandates say no one can predict a patient's future needs, but if that argument were taken to its logical endpoint, every insurance policy would cover every possible test and procedure and would be prohibitively expensive.

There is an indirect correlation between the number of mandates in any given state and the number of insurance policies per company offered in that state. Mandates restrict competition, drive up prices, and greatly restrict choices for patients. Although they have their place in medical treatment, not everyone wants or needs such things as acupuncture and chiropractic care.

Mandates are a classic example of politically powerful lobby groups forcing legislators to include their services with every insurance policy. They must be eliminated or severely restricted.

A reasonable first step would be to allow the interstate commerce of health care insurance. In other words, patients could purchase any approved insurance plan from any company in any state and pay for only those mandates dictated by the state of registration of that company. Literally overnight, patients would have a huge increase in their choices and the market would become much more competitive.

3) REFORM MEDICARE AND MEDICAID

Strong evidence exists that there was limited need for a non-means-tested socialized health insurance program for seniors at the time Medicare was implemented. As it came about with an increase in Social Security benefits, Medicare was a step along the path to completely socializing medicine in the United States.

Regardless of how it started, there is virtually complete agreement that Medicare is not financially sustainable in its present form. The costs are rising, the number of workers to support the program is proportionately decreasing, and the number of recipients is about to increase dramatically as the baby boomers approach age sixty-five.

We now have an entire generation that has grown up with Medicare, has paid into it, and expects something in return. We also have people in a younger generation that understand the bankrupt nature of the program and do not believe Medicare will exist when they reach age sixty-five.

So the solution to the Medicare problem must account for both of these generations, as well as future generations. We as a country have a moral obligation to those seniors already enrolled in the program and those approaching retirement. Simple first steps to unwinding Medicare would be to raise the age of eligibility to sixty-eight or seventy years and to require means testing for enrollment. And Medicare should be de-coupled from Social Security, so retirees can receive Social Security benefits even though they don't participate in Medicare.

As it stands now, there is, understandably, no private insurance market for seniors. This market could be resurrected by allowing people out of Medicare - currently they are a captive group of patients with no other alternatives.

Future generations should be allowed to take their individual health care insurance into retirement. No surprise, younger people as a group are healthier than older people, so as the younger generation saves, their health care insurance nest egg can build until they need it in their later years.

Transitioning Medicare from our current pay-as-you-go program of coverage for everyone to a program of individual choice would be very expensive and would undoubtedly require increased funding from the general tax revenue stream. Yet, the cost of the current Medicare program over the next thirty years will be extremely expensive as well, so why not spend that money transitioning to a program that will work and be sustainable?

Medicaid is in the same unsustainable financial condition as Medicare - perhaps worse. We cannot abandon the poor, but giving them mandated, unlimited, first-dollar coverage is both financially and ethically unsound. A voucher system allowing for personal choice and a financial reward for dollars saved would be an excellent start to unwinding the current Medicaid program.

States should also be able to get Medicaid waivers and receive block grants of money from the federal government. States could budget more efficiently with a fixed amount of money in a block grant rather than the open-ended entitlement nature of the current Medicaid program. States could also design their own innovative programs without rules and regulations from the federal government.

Strong consideration should be given to returning to the original income requirement of 133 percent of the federal poverty level for Medicaid recipients. In many states, Medicaid is now a "safety net" for people well into the middle economic class.

4) ENACT TORT REFORM

Nearly 20 percent of our health care budget is spent on the legal system through attorneys' fees, court costs, malpractice insurance premiums, and most importantly, defensive medicine practices. Medical outcomes in the U.S. are no worse, and in many ways much better, than other countries, yet our legal system burdens our health care spending much more than the legal systems other countries have in place. This must stop.

States that have enacted meaningful tort reform now enjoy a greater choice of physicians and have all specialties available to their citizens. Every patient in those states still has access to the legal system, but medical overhead is significantly less. Texas is but one example. Since passage of tort reform legislation in 2003, Texas has seen an influx of 4,000 physicians per year and malpractice premiums for doctors have decreased from thirteen to twenty-two percent depending on the physician's specialty (Gingrich and Gill, 2006).

Regardless of whether tort reform is a states-rights issue, it must be done in every state. Meaningful caps on non-economic damages offer the main solution to our current legal award lottery.

5) MAKE HEALTH 'INSURANCE' TRUE INDEMNITY INSURANCE

We also need a fundamental change in how we view health insurance. Instead of this "insurance" covering every health-related activity, it needs to work like other forms of indemnity insurance such as car and homeowners insurance.

Just as no one uses insurance to pay for gas or to mow the lawn, we need to get away from the idea of health insurance covering all our health-related events. True indemnity insurance should be there for catastrophes and emergencies. Day to day things should be paid for out of pocket.

A terrific mechanism to do this today is through the use of a health savings account (HSA). These accounts require a person or family to purchase a high-deductible catastrophic policy, but allow a tax-advantaged savings account for day-to-day medical-related purchases. Savings can be rolled over from year to year and can be taken from one job to another. For example, if a family has a five-thousand-dollar deductible but only spends two thousand in one year, they can roll the other three thousand dollars into next year's account.

The number of people using HSAs grows each year. Satisfaction is extremely high and medical outcomes are comparable to people with first-dollar-coverage health insurance. Health care related expenses for people with HSAs are proving to be much less than for people with traditional insurance.

Expanding the use of HSAs, even to patients over the age of sixty-five, would go a long way to establishing a real insurance system in health care. HSAs would increase patient choice and control and would ultimately make the patient a more informed consumer. Patients, as health care consumers, would demand more transparency in pricing and, just like in other economic areas, would force competition, improve quality and drive costs down.

19.
CONCLUSION

So let's go back to our food discussion. Everyone in this country has a right to decide what kind and how much food they want and need. Everyone understands they are financially responsible for obtaining their own food. Everyone has a right to *access* food, not a right to free food paid for partially or completely by someone else.

Health care and food care do not need to be treated differently. No one believes we should socialize our food delivery system, yet this same reasoning eludes many people when they think about health care.

Our current health delivery system is not financially sustainable. A true free market should be created where patients, as consumers, are allowed to select the type and amount of care they want and need. The government's responsibility should be to provide the structure for the free market to exist.

The socialized, government-run programs of Medicare and Medicaid are in severe financial trouble and have been fiscally unsound since their inception. It is absolutely foolhardy to believe that more government intervention in the form of the new health care law (PPACA) or completely socialized care would be more financially solvent. Quite simply, we cannot afford complete and total universal health care.

Furthermore, our country is based on free choice, and this philosophy needs to be applied to the medical area of our lives as well. The rationing, the lack of patient control, and the wage and price fixing that accompany socialized health care are totally at odds with this country's underlying beliefs. Only through massive reform of our current system will we be able to allow patients and health care providers the free market format to interact and individualize care as needed.

CITED REFERENCES

Adams, Scott J. 2004. Employer-provided health insurance and job change. *Contemporary Economic Policy,* 2004. 22 (3): 357–369.

Bureau of the Census. *Historical statistics of the United States: Colonial times to 1970,* Bicentennial Edition Part 1. Washington, DC: Government Printing Office, 1975.

Califano, Jr., Joseph A. *American health care revolution.* New York: Random House, 1986, pg. 41.

Cannon, Michael F. and M. D. Tanner. *Healthy competition.* Washington, DC: Cato Institute, 2005, pg. 116.

Cantril, Hadley. Public opinion 1935–1946. Princeton: Princeton University Press, 1951, pgs. 442–443.

Carson, Gerald. *The personal income tax: Where it came from, how it grew.* Boston: Houghton Mifflin, 1977, pgs. 12–129.

Congressional Budget Office, How many people lack health insurance and for how long? CBIO, Washington, DC. May 2003.

Conover, Christopher. Health care regulations: A $169 billion tax. Cato Institute *Policy Analysis no. 527*, October 4, 2004.

Contract practice. *Journal of the American Medical Association*, 1907. 49: 2028–2029.

Contract practice. *Journal of the American Medical Association*, 1911. 57: 145–146.

Danzon, Patricia M. Hidden overhead costs: Is Canada's system really less expensive? *Health Affairs*, 1992. 11(1): 21–43.

Editorial Page, "Mitt's Non-Miracle." *Wall Street Journal*, May 2, 2006.

Ezrati, Milton. "Medicare and the Federal Budget." *Lord Abbett's Economic Insights*, http://www.lordabbett.com/us/home.jsp, January 16, 2004.

Feingold, Eugene. *Medicare: Policy and politics*. San Francisco: Chandler Publishing Company, 1966, pgs. 91–92.

German Health Care, http://www.dw-world.de/dw/article/ 0.22144.1973312.00.html, accessed June 2007.

Gingrich, Newt and J. T. Gill, "Prodigal State." *Wall Street Journal*, May 4, 2006.

Harris, Richard. *A sacred trust*. New York: The New American Library, 1966, pg. 9.

Hayward, Rodney A. and T. P. Hofer. 2001. Estimating hospital deaths due to medical errors: Preventability is in the eye of the reviewer. *Journal of the American Medical Society,* 2001. 286: 415–420.

Health care in Canada. Ottawa: Canadian Institute for Health Information, 2004, pg. 42.

Henderson, David. *Better medicine: Reforming Canadian health care.* Montreal: ECW Press, 2002, pgs. 177–178.

Japan Health Care, http://www.sq.ernb-japan.gojp/ JapanAccess//health.htm, accessed June 2007.

Kling, Arnold. "Bill of Health." *Wall Street Journal*, April, 7, 2006.

Moon, Marilyn. Testimony before the U.S. Senate Committee on Finance, May 27, 1999.

Newhouse, Joseph P. and the Insurance Experimental Group. *Free for all? Lessons from the RAND Health Insurance Experiment.* Cambridge, Mass: Harvard University Press, 1996.

Organization for Economic Cooperation and Development. *Infant mortality, deaths per 1,000 live births.* OCED Health Data 2004, third edition.

Pearman, William A. and P. Starr. *Medicare: A handbook on the history and issues of health care services for the elderly.* New York: Garland Publishing, 1988, pg.23.

Pardes, Herbert, "The Coming Doctor Shortage." *Wall Street Journal,* January 19, 2011.

Price Waterhouse Coopers, *The Factors Fueling Rising Health Care Costs.* Washington, D.C., April, 2002.

Reinhardt, Uwe E., P. S. Hussey, and G. F. Anderson. 2004. U.S. health care spending in an international context. *Health Affairs,* 2004. 23(3): 11–12.

Ricardo-Campbell, Rita. *The economics and politics of health care.* Chapel Hill: University of North Carolina Press, 1982, pg. 93.

Starr, Paul. *The social transformation of American medicine.* New York: Basic Books, 1982, pg. 311.

Stern, Martha. "Medicare: Diagnosis Grim, Prognosis Grimmer." *Wall Street Journal,* June 4, 1991.

Tanner, Michael. The Grass is Not Always Greener: A Look At National Health Care Systems Around the World. CATO Press, Washington, D.C., March, 2008.

U.S. Senate Committee on Finance (89-1), *Social Security: Hearings* (On H.R. 6675), April/May 1965, pg. 818.

United States Department of Health and Human Services. *Improper fiscal year 2000 Medicare fee-for-service payments.* Report A-17-00-02000, March 6, 2001.

Wesley, Terre P. *What has government done to our health care?* Washington, DC: Cato Institute, 1992, pgs. 56–57.

Yelowitz, Aaron and Cannon, Michael. *"The Massachusetts Health Plan: Much Pain, Little Gain".* Washington, D.C.: CATO Institute, January, 2010.

REFERENCES FOR FIGURES

Figure 1

Bureau of the Census, *Historical statistics of the United States: Colonial times to 1970, Bicentennial edition, part 1*. Washington, D.C.: Government Printing Office, 1975.

Bureau of the Census, *Statistical abstract of the United States, 1996*. Washington, D.C.: Government Printing Office, 1996.

Katharine Levit et al. 2000. Health spending in 1998: Signals of change. *Health Affairs*, 2000. 19(1).

Center for Medicare and Medicaid Services. 2010 Health Care Statistics. Washington, D.C., 2010.

Figure 2

Dale H. Gieringer. 1985. The safety and efficacy of new drug approval. *Cato Journal* 5(1), pgs. 177–201.

Figure 3

U.S. Senate Committee on Finance. *Social Security*, hearings on H.R. 6675, April–May, 1965.

Social Security Administration. *Social Security: Facts and figures.* SSA publication 05-10011, May 1997.

Figure 4

Andrew J. Rettenmaier and Thomas R. Saving. The 2009 Annual Report of the Boards of Trustees of the Federal Hospital Insurance and Federal Supplemental Medical Insurance Trust Funds. *National Center for Policy Analysis Policy Report, 2009*

Figure 5

Marilyn Moon, of the Urban Institute. Medicare matters: The value of social insurance. Testimony before the U.S. Senate Committee on Finance, May 27, 1999

Figure 6

Centers for Medicare & Medicaid Services, Office of the Actuary, Table 1: National health expenditures and selected economic indicators, levels and average percent change: Selected calendar years 1990–2013. September 17, 2004.

The 2005 annual report of the board of trustees of the federal old age and survivors insurance and disability insurance trust funds. Washington, D.C.: Government Printing Office. March 23, 2005, pg. 60.

World Development Indicators database. Total GDP 2004. World Bank. July 2005, pg. 4.

The 2005 annual report of the board of trustees of the federal hospital insurance and federal supplementary medical insurance trust funds. Washington, D.C.: Government Printing Office. March 23,

2005, pgs. 64, 102, and 113.

Villareal, Pamela. *Social Security and Medicare Projections: 2009*. National Center for Policy Analysis. June 11, 2009.

Figure 7

National Association of State Budget Officers. *2003 state expenditure report*. October 2004, pgs. 16, 47, and 49.http://www.statehealthfacts.org/comparecat.jsp?cat=4

Figure 8

D.Eric Schansberg, *Cato Journal*, 31(1), Winter 2011, CATO Institute, Washington, D.C.

Figure 9

2003 Data Compendium, Centers for Medicare & Medicaid Services. National health care source of funds, selected calendar years. November 2003.

GENERAL REFERENCES

Bennett, James T. and T. J. Di Lorenzo. *From pathology to politics.* New Brunswick: Transaction Publishers, 2000.

Blevins, Sue A. *Medicare's midlife crisis.* Washington, D.C.: Cato Institute, 2001.

Cannon, Michael F. and M. D. Tanner. *Healthy competition. Second Edition,* Washington, D.C.: Cato Institute, 2007.

Friedman, Milton and Rose. *Free to choose.* New York: Harcourt Brace Jovanovich, Inc., 1980.

Goodman, John C. and G. L. Musgrave. *Patient power.* Washington, D.C.: Cato Institute, 1994.

Graham, John R. *What states can do to reform health care: A free market primer.* Pacific Research Institute, 2006.

Gratzer, David. *The cure.* New York: Encounter Books, 2006.

Sowell, Thomas. *Basic economics.* New York: Basic Books, 2000.

Wasley, Terree P. *What has government done to our health care?* Washington, D.C.: Cato Institute, 1992.

ABOUT THE AUTHOR

Dr. Roger Stark is a health care policy analyst at WPC and a retired physician. He is the author of numerous in-depth studies on health care policy, including *State Abuse of the Medicaid Program, A Review of the Medicaid Program: Its Impact in Washington State and Efforts at Reform in Other States, What Works and What Doesn't: A Review of Health Care Reform in the States*, and *Health Care Reform that Works: An Update on Health Savings Accounts*. After practicing in Tacoma he moved to Bellevue and was one of the co-founders of the open heart surgery program at Overlake Hospital. He retired from private practice in 2001 and became actively involved in the hospital's Foundation, serving as Board Chair and Executive Director. He is a past member of the hospital's Governing Board. Dr. Stark has been a member of many local and national professional societies.

Washington Policy Center (WPC) is an independent, non-profit, think tank that promotes sound public policy based on free-market solutions. WPC improves lives of Washington state's citizens by providing accurate, high-quality research for policymakers, the media and the general public.

Headquartered in Seattle, with offices in Olympia and Eastern Washington, WPC publishes studies, sponsors events and conferences and educates citizens on the vital public policy issues facing our region. WPC has an annual budget of $2 million and a full-time staff of 16. Broadcast, print, and online media throughout Washington and across the nation cover WPC's work regularly and seek out its policy experts for analysis and commentary. In addition, lawmakers routinely invite WPC to testify before legislative committees.

14237436R00078

Made in the USA
Lexington, KY
15 March 2012